J.J. Archer

RunShift™:

A Simple 5-Gear Method for 5K, 10K, and Half Marathon Success

Contact and info: jjarcherrunning.com

RunShift™: A <u>Simple</u> 5-Gear Method for 5K, 10K, and Half Marathon Success

Contents

Preface: Why I Wrote This Guide

Running has been one of the great constants of my life. Through different decades, jobs, challenges, and joys, lacing up and heading out the door has always been there for me. Now, in my sixties, I still run five days a week. I've raced marathons around the world, collected a wall of medals, and logged more miles than I can count. But the truth is, my favorite runs are often the half marathons I do quietly, on my own.

What running has taught me is simple: progress doesn't come from magic formulas or complicated charts. It comes from rhythm, patience, and learning to listen to your body. Over the years I devoured training books, searching for wisdom, but too often they buried good advice under jargon and theory. I wanted a way to make running easier to understand, not harder.

That search became a mission. I started sharing what I had learned with friends, family, and runners I met and coached along the way. I trained with them, encouraged them, and showed them the simple habits that work. The response was always the same: *"You should write this down."* What felt natural to me — clear, simple, practical advice — turned out to be exactly what others needed.

This book is my answer to those voices. As a friend of mine put, "Finally, a running method that's simple enough to follow and powerful enough to work."

RunShift™ is a method built on years of experience and countless miles. It is straightforward, adaptable, and designed for runners of all ages and levels. My promise to you is that this book contains all you need to know, and nothing you don't. It will help you run smarter, stay injury-free, and discover the joy of progress — whether your goal is a first 5K, a personal best, or simply to keep running for life.

Here it is: a lifetime of running, distilled into a system of gears you can use not just for training, but for the journey ahead.

Introduction: Why RunShift™

Most running plans fail for one of two reasons: they are either too complicated or too rigid. Many guides are filled with jargon, technical charts, and conflicting advice that leave runners confused before they even start. Others oversimplify, pushing a "one-speed-fits-all" model that quickly leads to burnout, injury, or boredom.

The RunShift Method™ is built on a simple but powerful idea: your body runs like an engine with gears. Instead of rigid charts or formulas, you learn to shift smoothly between five gears — from easy cruise to full sprint — depending on the purpose of each run. This makes training flexible, intuitive, and sustainable. Whether you're chasing your first 5K or refining your half- marathon, the RunShift Method™ helps you run smarter, stay consistent, and enjoy the process, because progress comes not from grinding harder, but from shifting at the right time.

RunShift™: A <u>Simple</u> 5-Gear Method for 5K, 10K, and Half Marathon Success

Running has become a major focus of sports science, and with it has come a flood of data that can leave runners confused and overwhelmed. What exactly is my lactate threshold? Is it tied to my maximum heart rate (and how do I even know that)? The old "220 minus your age" formula is notoriously imprecise and often inaccurate (too high or too low). And then there's functional thresholds like VO_2 max, and more. The RunShift Method™ is grounded in science so

Sports science has given us a flood of metrics, each with its own formula and debate:

- **Lactate threshold** – *the effort where lactic acid starts building up faster than your body can clear it.*
- **Maximum heart rate** – *often estimated as 220 minus your age, but this rule of thumb can be far off.*
- **Functional threshold** – *the maximum pace or power you could sustain for about an hour.*
- **VO_2 max** – *a lab-based measure of how much oxygen your body can use.*

*Useful for researchers and elite athletes, but confusing for most runners. The **RunShift Method™** distills the science into something simple: shift gears by feel (see chapter 2), not formulas.*

you don't have to chase every metric. All you need to do is learn to shift, enjoy your runs, and watch your progress unfold.

Runners who progress the most, and enjoy the process, are those who learn to shift.

The Promise of RunShift™

The RunShift™ method is built around one promise: learn the gears, train smarter, and enjoy running more.

Instead of complicated training zones or endless math, you'll learn to think of your body as an engine with gears. Each gear has a purpose, and by shifting between them, you'll build endurance, strength, speed, and resilience in a way that feels natural and sustainable.

The RunShift Method: Better than Heartrate

Think of driving a stick-shift car or riding a motorcycle. You don't stay in one gear the entire ride. You shift up to cruise, down to climb a hill, and back to neutral when you stop. Each gear has its role, and together they make the ride smooth, powerful, and efficient.

Running works the same way. Your body has "gears": different speeds, different intensities, different purposes. By learning how to use them, you can train with purpose, avoid burning out, and actually enjoy the process of getting stronger.

The important thing to understand is this: gears are about how you feel — not about your heartrate.

Many training plans try to lock runners into heart-rate zones. While heart-rate training can be useful, it's often confusing and frustrating because heartrate is influenced by so many factors:

- **Fatigue:** A tired runner may see elevated heartrates even at easy paces.
- **Temperature and humidity:** Heat drives your heartrate up, even if your effort stays the same.
- **Stress or lack of sleep:** Both can raise your resting and training heartrates.

- **Age and fitness level:** Maximum heartrates vary widely between individuals, and formulas are often unreliable.
- **Terrain.** Your heart rate will naturally go up during a climb.

This means that two runners running side by side (or even the same runner on different day) could see very different heart-rate numbers for the same effort.

That's why the RunShift method is simpler and more reliable. It's **feel-based**: you measure your effort by your breathing, your ability to talk, and your sense of sustainability. These cues are always with you, and they adjust naturally to your fitness, the weather, and how you feel on that day.

By focusing on gears instead of heartrate, you take the guesswork and variability caused by many factors out of training. You don't need lab equipment or complex formulas, just awareness of your body. The gears put you in control, every time you lace up.

The RunShift Method: Better than Pace

Pace, like heart rate, is highly variable. Environmental factors such as heat, humidity, or headwinds can slow you down, and for women, hormonal changes across the menstrual cycle can also influence performance. These fluctuations are normal and temporary. The encouraging news is that as you train, your body adapts (increasing capillary density, mitochondrial efficiency, and fuel utilization), so *your pace at the same gear will improve.* That's why the RunShift™ method provides a more accurate and sustainable guide.

Your effort, not your pace, should stay roughly consistent. I once ran with a friend who braked all the way down a hill because his watch kept beeping when he exceeded his target pace. That's a perfect example of why I prefer training by gears instead of numbers. When the terrain gives you free speed, take it! As long as the slope is safe, let gravity do the work. Likewise, don't fight the hills and expect your pace to drop on the way up. Running at the same pace uphill and downhill doesn't feel the same, *because it isn't the same.* It is entirely normal to run slightly lower when going uphill and slightly faster when going downhill.

Because your pace will vary at any given gear, I recommend not focusing on it too much. If you wear a sports watch, try not to check it constantly. Better yet, adjust the display so it doesn't show your current pace at all. If you like, you can keep average pace visible, or simply review your data after the run. What matters most is learning to recognize your gears using the simple tests explained in Chapter 2.

The Gears of Running

- **Neutral:** Walking. Your recovery and reset mode, the foundation of rest.
- **Gear 1:** Very slow running. Conversational, fully comfortable.
- **Gear 2:** The main training gear. Steady, sustainable, and the heart of your running.
- **Gear 3:** Tempo running. Challenging but controlled.
- **Gear 4:** Fast intervals. Hard effort you can sustain for only a few minutes.
- **Gear 5:** Sprinting. Short bursts at maximum effort.

By shifting between these gears, you'll train every part of your "engine": endurance, strength, speed, and efficiency. The method gives structure and variety to your training without requiring advanced science degrees or expensive technology. It's practical, memorable, and effective.

Why Gears Make Sense

Most runners get stuck in the wrong gear(s):

- Beginners often run too hard, quickly burning out or getting injured.
- More experienced runners sometimes stay too comfortable, never pushing into the gears that unlock new progress.

The RunShift™ method solves both problems. It shows you when to hold back, when to push, and when to recover, all by shifting gears like a driver in control of their vehicle.

With this method, you'll learn not just how to run, but how to run well. Training becomes less about confusion or struggle, and more about rhythm and flow. Once you master your gears, running is no longer something you grind through; it's a skill you can enjoy for a lifetime.

Using the Gears on a Treadmill

Can you use the RunShift™ method on a treadmill? Absolutely! I lived in the Southeastern U.S. for many years, and running outside in July and August was often unpleasant, even unbearable at times. The treadmill became my training partner, and the RunShift method translate perfectly indoors.

Each gear corresponds to a specific pace, which is easy to set on a treadmill. To make the effort closer to outdoor running, I recommend adding a **0.5% incline**. This small adjustment helps mimic wind resistance and natural terrain.

Tip: Many treadmills come with built-in programs or coaching features. They may not match the workouts in Chapters 10 and 11 exactly, but if they keep you motivated, use them. Just check in with yourself and *note which gear you're in.* Thinking in gears makes it easy to translate treadmill sessions to outdoor runs.

For longer treadmill runs, I like to watch videos of coaches running through scenic landscapes (shout-out to Tommy Rivs!). That visual link to the outdoors makes the miles feel less confined. If your treadmill has an auto-adjust mode, use caution. Sudden pace changes often don't line up with RunShift workouts, especially on interval days. On those days, I prefer setting my own speed and simply playing the videos for scenery.

Movies or sports broadcasts can also help the time pass, but avoid anything too intense. Action scenes or high-stakes games can spike your adrenaline. Save that for race day!

Remember: the treadmill is another tool in your toolbox. Use it to stay consistent, whatever the weather brings.

RunShift™: A <u>Simple</u> 5-Gear Method for 5K, 10K, and Half Marathon Success

---

Pro Tips for Treadmill Training

Built-in programs: Many treadmills offer coaching features or preset workouts. Use them if they keep you motivated. Just check your effort and adjust the pace to the right gear.

Scenic videos: Long treadmill sessions feel easier with landscape videos or coach-led runs. They add a sense of connection to the outdoors.

Smart entertainment: Movies or sports can help pass the time, but avoid adrenaline-heavy action — save that surge for race day.

Using the Gears When You're Out of Shape

If you feel that running isn't for you because you're "starting from too far back," don't worry. The gear system is designed to meet you exactly where you are. You'll find guidance in Chapter 10 on how to make small adjustments to the training plans later in this guide so you can build fitness safely and gradually.

◆ **Key Takeaway:** Other plans confuse or oversimplify. RunShift™ simplifies without dumbing down — giving you a clear, flexible method you can use to run smarter, stay consistent, and love the process.

Part I. The RunShift™ Method

Chapter 1. Understanding the Five Gears

An Important Word of Caution Before You Start

Running is one of the simplest and most rewarding ways to get fit, but it is still a form of physical stress. Before starting a new exercise program, or making significant changes to your current one, it's best to consult with a physician or qualified health professional. This is especially important if you have existing health conditions, are returning from injury, or have been inactive for a long period.

During your runs, always listen to your body. If you experience **sharp or significant pain, dizziness, chest tightness, or unusual shortness of breath**, stop immediately and seek medical guidance. Discomfort from effort is normal; pain that feels alarming is not. Running should challenge you, but it should never put your health at risk.

Why Gears Matter

When you drive a stick-shift car or ride a motorcycle, you don't stay in the same gear all the time. Each gear has its purpose: starting smoothly, cruising comfortably, accelerating with power, or sprinting to top speed. Running works the same way. The secret to training well isn't running harder all the time; it's learning when and how to "shift" into the right gear.

The RunShift™ method[1] organizes running into five gears plus neutral, each with its own role. Mastering these gears will not only make you a smarter runner but also help prevent overtraining, burnout, and injury. Let's walk through them.

I call the second gear the *natural* gear. Evolutionary biologists such as Dennis Bramble and Daniel Lieberman (see box on the right and, if you want to learn more, Appendix D) have argued that humans are uniquely adapted for endurance running. Our ancestors often covered long distances under the sun, sometimes while persistence hunting, and likely did so while communicating with others in their group. Gear 2 reflects that deep evolutionary design: it is steady, sustainable, and built for conversation. It is the gear your body was made to use for longer runs — the foundation on which everything else rests.

---

[1] "Shift" refers to moving through gears of effort; it is not about forcing a lean forward at all times, which some people may refer to as "shift running."

Neutral Gear: Walking

- **Purpose:** Recovery.
- **How it feels:** Relaxed. Your heartrate is low, and breathing is easy.
- **When to use it:** During warm-ups, cooldowns, recovery between intervals, and recovery days.
- **Why it matters:** Walking lets your body circulate blood, carry away waste products, and reset without shutting down completely. Think of it as idling at a stoplight: the engine is still on, but you're not pushing it.

Gear 1: The (Very) Easy Gear

- **Purpose:** Active recovery.
- **How it feels:** You can chat easily with a friend or even talk on the phone without gasping. If necessary, especially if you're out of shape, it is perfectly fine to walk in Gear 1.
- **Test:** Full conversation is possible.
- **Training role:** Use this gear to recover from harder runs while still logging gentle miles. It's also the gear you can use occasionally when you're just getting started as a runner.
- **Why it matters:** This is the foundation of your running "engine." Skipping Gear 1 and always pushing harder is like redlining your car every time you drive. Eventually, something breaks.

RunShift™: A <u>Simple</u> 5-Gear Method for 5K, 10K, and Half Marathon Success

Evolutionary biologists Dennis Bramble and Daniel Lieberman have shown that the human body carries unique adaptations for endurance running. Unlike most primates, we:

Cool efficiently: Millions of sweat glands and little body hair let us shed heat while moving.

Store and use energy well: Our bodies can switch between fat and glycogen to keep going for hours.

Run smoothly: Spring-like tendons (Achilles, plantar arch) store energy; large gluteus muscles and a stabilizing nuchal ligament keep us upright and balanced.

Communicate on the move: Our ability to breathe rhythmically and still talk made it possible to coordinate during long runs, hunts, or migrations.

Anthropologists call this the endurance running hypothesis: that humans survived and thrived in part because we could outlast prey and cover long distances together.

When you run in Gear 2, you're tapping into this ancient design. It feels natural because it is natural: a gear honed over hundreds of thousands of years. That's why it should form the heart of your training today.

Gear 2: The Natural Gear

- **Purpose:** The workhorse of your training. 70–80% of all your runs should be here.
- **How it feels:** Comfortable but steady. You could keep going for a long time, but you're aware you're running. *If you're feeling a pinch, you're no longer in Gear 2.*
- **Test:** You can still talk, but the conversation has pauses.
- **Training role:** Long runs, weekly base runs, warmups, and cooldowns.
- **Why it matters:** Gear 2 builds aerobic capacity, which is the ability to use oxygen efficiently. This is what makes marathons possible, helps you run longer without fatigue, and keeps training sustainable.

Gear 3: Tempo Gear

- **Purpose:** Improve your ability to sustain speed over longer distances.
- **How it feels:** You're working, but definitely not all-out. It feels "comfortably hard."
- **Test:** Talking is limited to short bursts or single words.
- **Training role:** Important but used sparingly in training. Critical for races. It often mirrors the effort of a half marathon or 10K.

- **Why it matters:** Gear 3 is where you train your body and mind to stay strong when things get uncomfortable. It's the bridge between cruising and really pushing.

Gear 4: Interval Gear

- **Purpose:** Develop speed and strength.
- **How it feels:** Hard. Your breathing is heavy, and you can only keep this pace for a few minutes.
- **Test:** You could say a few words, but you'd rather not.
- **Training role:** Used in long interval workouts, for example, sets of 2 minutes at Gear 4, with recovery in lower gears.
- **Why it matters:** Gear 4 teaches your body to handle fatigue, improve lactate threshold, and sustain faster speeds. It's like hitting the gas to merge onto the highway: short, powerful efforts.

Gear 5 — Sprint Gear

- **Purpose:** Maximum effort for short bursts.
- **How it feels:** You're running almost as fast as you can but still with control — as if you could push just a little harder if you had to (say, if a bear were chasing you).
- **Test:** Talking is basically impossible.

- **Training role:** Use Gear 5 only for short intervals (15–30 seconds) followed by longer recoveries.
- **Why it matters:** Sprint work improves running economy, stride power, and neuromuscular coordination. It is fine-tuning your engine for peak performance.

Tip: Shifting straight from first or second to fifth gear is a big jump. Move through Gear 3 for a few seconds before engaging Gear 5. It helps your body transition smoothly and safely into top speed.

Bringing It Together

Each gear has its place. Neutral and Gears 1–2 keep you steady for longer, Gear 3 teaches resilience, Gear 4 builds power, and Gear 5 adds sharpness. ***A good runner isn't someone who runs fast all the time; it's someone who knows when to shift.***

By practicing each gear, you'll gain control over your pace, learn your body's signals, and build confidence in any running situation. From your first 5K to a half marathon, RunShift™ gives you the toolkit to train like a driver who knows exactly when to change gears.

The Science Behind the Gears

At its core, running is about how your body produces and uses energy. Different gears recruit your muscles, lungs, and heart in different ways. The magic of the RunShift™ method is that by rotating through the gears, you train *all* of these systems without burning yourself out

- Aerobic vs. Anaerobic Energy
    - **Aerobic** means "with oxygen." This is your body's efficient energy system, powering you during Gears 1 and 2. It burns mostly fat and a steady trickle of carbohydrates. The payoff? You can go for hours.
    - **Anaerobic** means "without oxygen." This system kicks in at higher gears (4 and 5), when your muscles need energy faster than your body can supply it with oxygen. It's powerful, but it can only last for short bursts because it produces lactate and fatigue.
- **Heartrate and VO$_2$ Max**
  Exercise scientists often describe gears in terms of **heartrate zones** or **VO$_2$ max** (your body's maximum ability to use oxygen). But don't worry: you don't need lab tests to run well. As explained in the Introduction, so many factors affect heartrate. Each gear has a purpose.

- o **Gear 1 & 2:** aerobic base building.
  - o **Gear 3:** teaching your body to manage lactate.
  - o **Gear 4:** sharpening your ability to push near your limits.
  - o **Gear 5:** maximum recruitment of muscles, sprint economy.

- Think of it like this: Gears 1 and 2 build the size of your "engine," while Gears 3–5 tune the engine so it can handle higher speeds and surges. Both are essential, but in very different doses.

Why Most Runs Belong in Gear 2

One of the hardest lessons for runners — especially beginners — is that **easy running is not "wasted running."** In fact, most of your improvement will come from the comfortable miles, not the lung-burning ones. Anthropologists argue that traits we take for granted like our ability to sweat, our upright posture, and the big gluteus maximus that stabilizes us make humans uniquely capable of endurance running. This evolutionary background explains why Gear 2 running feels so natural: our species was built to cruise steadily for hours.

When you run in Gear 2, several key adaptations happen:

1. **Capillaries grow:** These tiny blood vessels increase, delivering more oxygen to your muscles.
2. **Mitochondria multiply:** These are the "power plants" in your cells. More mitochondria = more efficient energy use.
3. **Fat metabolism improves:** Your body learns to burn fat as fuel, saving precious glycogen for when you really need it.In plain English: the more you train in Gear 2, the longer and faster you'll be able to run *later* without hitting the wall.

When Gear 2 Feels Hard

If Gear 2 doesn't feel natural yet, alternate gently between Gears 1 and 2 during your runs. Start with one minute in Gear 1 and one minute in Gear 2, then increase the time spent in Gear 2 as it becomes more comfortable. Walking in Gear 1 is fine. The goal is to keep the effort enjoyable so you can build consistency and ease your way into longer stretches of running.

The Role of the Higher Gears

So, if Gear 2 is king, why bother with the higher gears? Because performance isn't just about endurance; it's also about speed, strength, and resilience.

- **Gear 3 (Tempo):** Think of this as teaching your body to *stay calm under pressure*. Scientifically, you're raising your "lactate threshold." That is the point at which fatigue chemicals start to build up in your blood. A higher threshold = you can run faster before you feel the burn.
- **Gear 4 (Intervals):** Here, you stress your cardiovascular system in controlled bursts. The science calls this "VO_2 max training," because it improves your body's maximum oxygen uptake. The result is more horsepower in your running engine.
- **Gear 5 (Sprints):** This isn't just about raw speed. Short sprints improve your **neuromuscular coordination**, which means basically, how efficiently your brain and muscles communicate. Even distance runners benefit because sprints fine-tune stride mechanics and leg power.

The Art of Shifting

The beauty of RunShift™ is that you don't need to obsess over numbers, graphs, or complicated workouts. You just need to know your gears, listen to your body, and shift with purpose.

- Use **Neutral and Gear 1** when you need recovery.
- Spend most of your time cruising in **Gear 2.**
- Sprinkle in **Gear 3** to build resilience.
- Tap into **Gear 4** to add sharpness and strength.
- Occasionally unleash **Gear 5** for pure power.

This balance (comfort most of the time, challenge some of the time) is what keeps runners improving year after year without burning out.

◆ **Key Takeaway:** Each gear trains a different part of your body's engine. Stay mostly in Gear 2, but don't forget to shift.

Chapter 2. How to Find Your Gears

Knowing the gears in theory is one thing; feeling them in your own body is another. Every runner is different. A pace that feels like Gear 2 for one person may feel like Gear 4 for someone else. That's why the RunShift™ method is built on *relative effort*, not rigid numbers.

Gears are feel-based, not heartrate, because too many factors affect heartrates, like fatigue, temperature and humidity, stress or lack of sleep and of course age and fitness level. Moreover, maximum heartrates vary widely between individuals, and formulas are often unreliable. This means that two runners running side by side (or even the same runner on different days) could see different heart-rate numbers for the same effort.

The good news? You don't need fancy lab equipment to find your gears. With a little practice, you can learn to shift smoothly by paying attention to your breathing, your ability to talk, and how your body feels (more about running equipment in chapter 9).

Try both the Talk Test and the Breath Test to determine which feels most natural for you. Once you find your preferred method, use the other occasionally to verify your gears and ensure your effort levels remain accurate.

The Talk Test

One of the oldest and simplest ways to gauge effort is the talk test. Just pay attention to how easily you can speak while running. And it's surprisingly accurate.

Neutral (Walking): Talking is effortless; you could recite poetry without strain.

Gear 1 (Easy Run): Full conversation is possible. You can chat with a running buddy or even take a phone call. (*For some runners, Gear 1 may simply be a brisk walk.*)

Gear 2 (Natural Gear): You can still talk in sentences, but with pauses for breath. A few lines, then a pause, then continue.

Gear 3 (Tempo): Talking shrinks to short bursts: just a few words at a time.

Gear 4 (Long intervals): You're limited to one or two words before gasping.

Gear 5 (Sprint): Talking is impossible; every ounce of focus is on breathing and effort.

If you can't say a few words in Gear 2, you're running too fast. The beauty of the talk test is that it adapts naturally to fitness level, weather, and fatigue. Your body is giving you the right feedback

The Breath Test

Another simple way to check which gear you're in is to pay attention to your breathing. Unlike heart-rate monitors or pace charts, your breath is always with you, and it gives instant feedback.

Here's how it lines up with the gears:

- **Neutral (Walking):** Breathing feels completely effortless.
- **Gear 1 (Easy Run):** Breathing is light and easy.
- **Gear 2 (Natural gear):** Breathing is steady and comfortable. You could breathe entirely through your nose if you wanted to, though mouth breathing is fine if that feels more natural.
- **Gear 3 (Tempo):** Nose breathing may still be possible for short stretches, but you'll likely switch to mouth breathing as the effort builds.
- **Gear 4 (Intervals):** Breathing is generally through the mouth and noticeably heavier. Try to keep it controlled — for example, count "2 in, 2 out" or "4 in, 4 out."
- **Gear 5 (Sprint):** Breathing is fast and hard through the mouth. It may feel chaotic, but don't forget to stay mindful and keep the air moving in and out.

How to Know Your Gear: Two Simple Tests

Gear	Talk Test	Breath Test
Neutral (Walking)	Talking is effortless; you could recite poetry.	Breathing is completely effortless.
Gear 1 (Easy Run or Brisk Walk)	Full conversation is easy; you could chat with a friend or on the phone.	Breathing is light and easy.
Gear 2 (Natural gear)	You can talk in sentences, but with pauses to breathe.	Steady, comfortable breathing; nose-only breathing possible (mouth if preferred).
Gear 3 (Tempo)	Talking is limited to short bursts, just a few words at a time.	Mostly mouth breathing; nose breathing only possible for short stretches.
Gear 4 (Intervals)	Only one or two words before gasping.	Heavy mouth breathing; keep it controlled (e.g., "2 in, 2 out" or "4 in, 4 out").
Gear 5 (Sprint)	Talking is impossible; all focus is on breathing and effort.	Fast, hard mouth breathing; feels chaotic — just keep the air moving.

You can also use tools like RPE or heart rate, but for most runners I've coached, they just aren't as simple or reliable as listening to your body.

The RPE Scale

Another tool you may have read about is the **Rate of Perceived Exertion (RPE)**. This is a 1–10 scale of how hard you feel you're working. I have always found it hard to apply. I found that people I was coaching would find it difficult to jump, from say a 3 to a 7 RPE. But if you know and like that system, the transition to the simpler RunShift™ method will be simple. Here are *approximate* conversions:

- **Neutral:** RPE 0–1 (effortless, strolling)
- **Gear 1:** RPE 2–3 (light effort, fully comfortable)
- **Gear 2:** RPE 4–5 (moderate, sustainable "forever pace")
- **Gear 3:** RPE 6–7 (comfortably hard, challenging but controlled)
- **Gear 4:** RPE 7–8 (hard, strong focus needed, only a few minutes sustainable)
- **Gear 5:** RPE 9–10 (maximum effort, full sprint, seconds only)

On some days, a certain pace mile might feel like RPE 4. On a hot, tired day, the same pace might feel like RPE 7. The key is to train the *effort*, not the number. But as you learn your gears, I believe you will find the RunShift™ method simpler and more straightforward.

Pace and Heartrate (Optional Tools)

For runners who love data, you can add pace or heartrate as cross-checks:

- **Pace:** Over time, you'll learn the pace ranges that match your gears. For example, if your Gear 2 pace is somewhere around 7:30 per kilometer (12:00 per mile), you'll start *recognizing* that rhythm. It will feel *natural.* But remember: pace is affected by terrain, weather, and fatigue, so don't rely on it alone because that 7:30 may well be 7:00 or less or 8:00 or more based on all those factors, but still be Gear 2.
- **Heartrate:** I don't encourage focusing on heart rate too much. Focus on your gears instead. I don't have my heartrate displayed on my watch when I run. I only look (sometimes) after a run. Many watches estimate heartrate zones. Here are ranges but treat them as a **rough guide only:**
    - Gear 1: 60–70% of max heartrate
    - Gear 2: 70–75%
    - Gear 3: 80–85%
    - Gear 4: 85–90%
    - Gear 5: 90–100%

But again, treat these as *approximate reference points*. Your body's signals are always the best guide. Use them if you're already used to this metric.

Learning by Practice

The first step in RunShift™ is simply to experiment. Don't worry about getting it perfect right away. With a little practice, you'll quickly learn to *feel* which gear you're in. Try this drill during your runs:

1. **Start Easy:** Warm up by walking in Neutral, then ease into Gear 1. Notice your breathing and how easy it is to hold a conversation.
2. **Cruise:** Shift up to Gear 2 and settle into a steady rhythm. Pay attention to how long you could comfortably maintain this pace.
3. **Push the Edge:** Move into Gear 3 for a few minutes, just enough to sense where comfort begins to turn into challenge. At some point in third gear, you will feel the run beginning to "pinch."
4. **Add Speed:** Try short bursts in Gears 4 and 5. Focus on how your stride, breathing, and concentration change at higher efforts.
5. **Recover:** Drop back down to Neutral or Gear 1 and notice how quickly your body settles.

These simple "gear drills" train your brain and body to connect effort with sensation. Within a few weeks, you'll begin to recognize your gears instinctively and shifting between them will feel natural.

Shifting as a Skill

Just like driving or riding a motorbike, shifting gears takes practice. At first, you'll over- or under-shoot. You'll find yourself running too fast in Gear 2 or holding back too much in Gear 4. That's normal. The more you practice, the smoother your shifts will become.

Eventually, you'll know your gears so well that you won't need to think about them. You'll just *feel* when it's time to downshift for recovery, hold steady in cruise mode, or rev up for a challenge. That's when running becomes second nature.

📌 **Key Takeaway:** Forget complicated lab tests. You already carry the best tools to gauge effort: your breath and your voice.

- **The Talk Test**: If you can talk in full sentences, you're in a low gear. If you can only say a few words,

you're working harder. If you can't speak at all, you're at the top.
- **The Breath Test**: Pay attention to rhythm. Smooth, even breathing = lower gears. Short, gasping breaths = high gears.

These simple checks adapt to weather, fatigue, and fitness level. They help you stay in the right gear no matter what the watch says.

With time, shifting becomes automatic, and running becomes more enjoyable and effective.

Chapter 3. Weekly Structure: 4-Day and 5-Day Runners

One of the biggest mistakes runners make is thinking that more is always better. More miles, more speed, more days. The truth is that progress comes not just from training, but from *balanced* training. Too much stress without recovery leads to fatigue, injury, or burnout. Too little challenge, and you plateau.

The RunShift™ method is designed for the sweet spot: training **four or five days a week**. This frequency is ideal for most recreational and intermediate runners. It's enough to make steady progress, but still leaves space for rest and recovery. Those are the days when your body actually adapts and gets stronger.

Why 4 or 5 Days?

- **Adaptation Time:** After a hard run, your muscles, tendons, and cardiovascular system need 24–48 hours to repair. Rest days aren't wasted days; they're where the improvements happen.
- **Injury Prevention:** Running every day dramatically increases stress on joints and connective tissues. Four to five days per week strikes a safe balance.

- **Consistency:** Most people can realistically commit to 4–5 runs. That consistency matters more than squeezing in extra mileage.

Elite athletes may train more often, but they also have years of base fitness, full-time support teams, and recovery routines most of us can't replicate. Your goal is *smart training, not maximum training.*

The Building Blocks of the Week

Every week in the RunShift™ method contains a **mix of gears**. Here's how it breaks down:

1. **The Long Run (Gear 2):** The cornerstone of your week. Builds endurance, mental strength, and aerobic capacity.
2. **The Basic Run (Gear 2, shorter):** Half the length of your long run. Reinforces endurance without overloading your body.
3. **The Interval Run:** Either long intervals (Gear 4) or short intervals (Gear 5), depending on the week. Develops speed, strength, and efficiency.
4. **The Optional Tempo Run (Gear 3):** For runners training 5 days a week, this is your fifth session. For 4-day runners, it replaces the long interval session once per month.

<u>4-Day Structure</u>

(note: chapter 11 contains a full 12-week plan based on this structure)

- **Day 1:** Long Run (Gear 2, see chapter 4)
- **Day 2:** Rest or active recovery
- **Day 3:** Basic Run (Gear 2, half the long run time. See chapter 5)
- **Day 4:** Rest or cross-training
- **Day 5:** Intervals (short or long, alternating weekly, See chapters 6 and 7)
- **Day 6:** Rest or easy walk/jog
- **Day 7:** Basic Run (Gear 2, steady)

Variation: Once a month, replace the long interval run with a Tempo Run (Gear 3. See chapter 8).

<u>5-Day Structure</u>

(note: chapter 11 contains a full 12-week plan based on this structure)

- **Day 1:** Long Run (Gear 2, see chapter 4)
- **Day 2:** Rest or active recovery
- **Day 3:** Basic Run (Gear 2, half the long run time. See chapter 5)
- **Day 4:** Intervals (long intervals, Gear 4. See chapter 6)
- **Day 5:** Rest or active recovery
- **Day 6:** Tempo Run (Gear 3. See chapter 8)
- **Day 7:** Short Intervals (sprints in Gear 5 with recovery in Gear 1. See chapter 7)

This extra day allows you to work all gears in the same week, with plenty of recovery time built in.

Active Recovery Days

Rest doesn't always mean doing nothing. Light activity on off days can help circulation and speed recovery. Examples include:

- Walking (Neutral gear)
- Gentle cycling or swimming
- Yoga or mobility work
- Pushups/planks
- Moderate weight/strength training

The key is that it should feel restorative, not strenuous.

Listening to Your Body

Schedules are important, but they're not set in stone. Some weeks, life will intervene. Other times, your body will tell you it needs more rest. That's not failure. It's smart training.

Signs you may need to swap a run for rest include:

- Persistent soreness or joint pain
- Trouble sleeping
- A sudden drop in motivation
- Elevated resting heartrate or unusual fatigue

Remember: running is a long game. Missing one session is never as damaging as pushing through and risking injury.

Stretching

Stretching is an excellent habit for runners. The best time depends on you. Personally, I prefer *not* to stretch *immediately after* a run because the muscle fibers are still "overexcited." Instead, I stretch later in the day, often in the evening.

At a minimum, I recommend focusing on **hamstrings, quadriceps, and calves**. Those are the three muscle groups that carry much of the load in your runs.

<u>Hamstrings</u>

- Lie on your back with one leg extended on the floor.
- Loop a belt or strap around the other foot and raise that leg straight up.
- Gently pull the leg toward you until you feel a stretch in the back of your thigh.
- Hold for 10 seconds, then pull a little farther. Hold again for another 10 seconds, and repeat once more.
- Keep the other leg on the ground as straight as possible throughout.

Quadriceps

This stretch is challenging at first, but well worth the effort.

- Kneel on the floor with your back against a door or wall, wearing clean shoes or thick slippers to protect the top of your foot.

- Place one foot up so the top of the foot rests flat against the wall or door.

- Step the other leg forward, raising the knee until it forms a 90-degree angle.
- Gradually lift your upper body toward the wall or door.
- At first you may not be able to get all the way upright, but within a couple of weeks it usually becomes easier.
- Hold for 30 seconds, then switch legs.

Calves

- Stand facing a wall, about two feet away.
- Place your hands on the wall and step one foot back.
- Keep the back heel pressed firmly into the ground and the back leg straight.
- Lean forward slightly until you feel a stretch along the calf of the back leg.
- Hold for 20–30 seconds, then switch sides.
- For a deeper stretch of the lower calf, repeat with the back knee bent.

With practice you can do all three stretches in a matter of a few minutes. These stretches are powerful tools for keeping your muscles loose and resilient. Just a few minutes of regular stretching can go a long way toward preventing stiffness, maintaining flexibility, and helping you feel stronger on your runs.

The Science of Variety

Why alternate gears instead of just running everything at one pace? Because variety triggers different adaptations:

- **Long Runs (Gear 2):** Build the aerobic engine, capillaries, and mitochondria.
- **Intervals (Gear 4 and 5):** Improve oxygen uptake (VO_2 max) and muscle recruitment.
- **Tempo Runs (Gear 3):** Raise lactate threshold, teaching your body to resist fatigue.

By combining these, you train the whole system: endurance, strength, and speed. That's how runners improve efficiently — without junk miles or wasted effort.

 Key Takeaway: Running four to five days a week with a balance of gears is the most effective way to train without burnout. Long runs build endurance, intervals build speed, and tempo runs build resilience — together they make you a stronger, smarter runner.

Chapter 4. The Long Run (Gear 2)

If there's one workout that defines RunShift™, it's the **long run**. This is the session that quietly builds endurance, teaches patience, and gives you the confidence to cover distances you once thought impossible. Ask any experienced runner: the long run is the backbone of training.

The long run connects us to our ancestors. Early humans may have used 'persistence hunting,' running animals to exhaustion under the sun. Today, you may be running for fitness or a half marathon, but physiologically it taps into the same ancient adaptation.

Why the Long Run Matters

The long run trains your body and mind in ways that shorter runs simply can't. Here's what happens when you spend extended time in **Gear 2**:

- **Capillary Growth:** Your body builds more tiny blood vessels to deliver oxygen to working muscles.

- **Mitochondrial Boost:** The "power plants" of your cells multiply, improving your ability to use energy efficiently.

The long run is more than mileage — it's the cornerstone of endurance.

- *Physiology: Long, steady sessions train your body to store more glycogen, build capillaries, and strengthen mitochondria — the "power plants" of your muscles. Over time, this makes every gear more efficient.*
- *Evolution: Anthropologists argue that early humans survived by covering long distances, often hunting by running animals to exhaustion. In many ways, the long run is our most natural form of training.*

That's why it deserves a central place in your week. Each long run builds not just stamina, but a deep connection to what your body was designed to do.

- **Fuel Adaptation:** Running longer teaches your body to burn fat as a primary fuel source, sparing glycogen for later. This is what prevents the dreaded "wall" in races.

- **Mental Endurance:** You practice being on your feet for an extended period, building confidence for race day.

Science aside, long runs teach one of the most important running lessons: **comfort is not the goal; sustainability is.**

Finding Your Long Run Pace

Your long run *is not a race.* It should be firmly in **Gear 2**, sometimes even brushing against Gear 1. If you find yourself breathing hard or struggling to talk, you're going too fast. Slow down. The goal is *time on your feet*, not speed.

How Long Should a Long Run Be? That depends on your target distance:

- **5K runners:** Long runs should be 30-50 minutes.
- **10K runners:** Long runs should be at least 60–90 minutes.
- **Half marathoners:** Long runs should be 75–120 minutes.

A good rule of thumb: increase your long run by **no more than 10% per week**. Every 3–4 weeks, scale back to a shorter long run to allow recovery. Think of it as two steps forward, one step back, a safer, more sustainable path to progress.

Tips for the Long Run

- **Fuel and Hydration:** Runs over 75 minutes often benefit from mid-run hydration. Beyond 90 minutes, consider bringing simple carbs (like gels, chews, or even a banana). Practice fueling in training so it feels natural in races.
- **Terrain:** Flat routes build steady endurance. Hilly routes add strength. Both are useful; rotate between them for variety.
- **Music or Podcasts:** Long runs are the one time where headphones can help. They make the time pass, especially if you run solo. Just keep the volume safe if you're running outdoors. More on this in chapter 9.
- **Mindset:** Break the run into chunks. Think "three 20-minute runs" instead of "one 60-minute run." It makes the distance feel less intimidating.

The "TBS" check:

On your long runs, take a moment every so often (for example, each time you hydrate) to do a quick "*Toes,*

Buttocks, and Shoulders" (TBS) check. Start with your toes: as your foot lands, they should feel like they're gently gripping the inside of your shoe. Then move to your buttocks, and think of them as your engine, driving you forward. If you run with a slight forward lean (which I like), let that lean come from the ankles, not the waist. Engaging your buttocks helps keep your posture tall and prevents you from bending at the hips. Glutes are important muscles for runners! Finally, check your shoulders: keep them relaxed but upright, with your head held high and eyes looking forward, not down. Use the mantra "Toes grip, butt drives, shoulders tall." to remember it

You can do a TBS check anytime, but it's especially valuable on long runs, when form often starts to slip. Practicing this habit will keep your stride efficient and reduce the risk of injury.

Common Mistakes

1. **Running too fast:** The most frequent error. Remember: Gear 2.
2. **Skipping long runs:** Consistency matters. Missed long runs are harder to make up than missed short ones.
3. **Ignoring recovery:** The day after a long run should almost always be rest or easy movement. That's when your body adapts.

Progression Examples

Here are sample 8-week long run progressions for different race goals. Adjust times up or down depending on your current fitness level. Intermediate and more advanced runners can definitely go longer. If you're feeling strong after the scheduled time, just keep going (except for recovery and taper week)! Chapter 11 contain full 12-week plans.

<u>For a 5K Goal</u>

Focus: building endurance beyond race distance to make 5K feel easy.

- Week 1: 15 min
- Week 2: 20 min
- Week 3: 30 min
- Week 4: 20 min (recovery week)
- Week 5: 30 min
- Week 6: 30 min
- Week 7: 35 min
- Week 8: 20 min (taper week)

RunShift™: A <u>Simple</u> 5-Gear Method for 5K, 10K, and Half Marathon Success

<u>For a 10K Goal</u>

Focus: extending endurance so 10K feels manageable, not overwhelming.

- Week 1: 35 min
- Week 2: 40 min
- Week 3: 50 min
- Week 4: 45 min (recovery week)
- Week 5: 50 min
- Week 6: 50 min
- Week 7: 55 min
- Week 8: 40 min (taper week)

<u>For a Half Marathon Goal</u>

Focus: preparing for sustained effort, building confidence for race day.

- Week 1: 60 min
- Week 2: 70 min
- Week 3: 80 min
- Week 4: 60 min (recovery week)
- Week 5: 90 min
- Week 6: 100 min
- Week 7: 110 min
- Week 8: 75 min (taper week)

Notice the rhythm: **gradual build, step back, build again, taper.** This structure trains endurance while reducing the risk of overtraining.

The Long Run as Ritual

For many runners, the long run becomes more than just a workout, it's a weekly ritual. A chance to disconnect from work, stress, and screens. Some call it moving meditation. Others use it as social time with a running partner. However you frame it, treat your long run as an anchor for your training week. Running to your own playlist can be a great addition (more on music and gear in chapter 9).

📌 **Key Takeaway:** The long run in Gear 2 is the foundation of endurance training. Run it slowly, build it gradually, and let it become your weekly ritual — whether your goal is a 5K, 10K, or half marathon.

Chapter 5. The Basic Run (Gear 2, Shorter)

If the long run is the cornerstone of your training week, the **basic run** is the supporting pillar. It doesn't grab attention with dramatic distances or high speeds, but it's just as important. The basic run is where you quietly build strength, reinforce endurance, and teach your body the rhythm of consistent running.

What Is a Basic Run?

The basic run is a shorter Gear 2 run, usually about <u>half the length of your weekly long run.</u>

- **Gear:** Always in Gear 2 (steady and sustainable).
- **Duration:** 20–60 minutes depending on your fitness level.
- **Effort:** Conversation pace steady breathing, comfortable rhythm.

It may feel too easy at first, **but that's the point.** Training isn't just about pushing limits; it's about accumulating *quality time at the right effort.*

Why the Basic Run Matters

1. **Reinforces Endurance:** While the long run stretches your limits, the basic run strengthens your base in manageable chunks. Think of it as layering bricks on an already strong foundation.
2. **Supports Recovery:** Gear 2 runs increase blood flow and help your muscles repair from harder sessions without adding too much strain.
3. **Builds Consistency:** It's easier to stay consistent with short runs. Over time, that consistency adds up.
4. **Mental Training:** Learning to run at a comfortable effort teaches pacing discipline, one of the most underrated skills in running.

From a scientific perspective, the adaptations are similar to the long run but achieved with less stress: more capillaries, stronger mitochondria, better fat metabolism.

How to Structure Your Basic Run

- **Warm Up:** 5–10 minutes in Gear 1 (easy jogging or brisk walking).
- **Main Run:** 5–40 minutes in Gear 2. If your long run is 1 hour, your basic run should be about 30 minutes. If your long run is 90 minutes, your basic run should be about 45 minutes.
- **Cool Down:** 5–10 minutes in Gear 1 or Neutral (walking).

That's it. No sprints, no intervals, no fancy tricks. Just steady running.

Progression Examples

Like the long run, the basic run should grow gradually as you advance:

- **5K Runners:** Start at 15 minutes. Build up over a training cycle.
- **10K Runners:** Start at 30 minutes. Build up to 45–50 minutes.
- **Half Marathon Runners:** Start at 35–40 minutes. Build up to 60 minutes.

Always remember the "half the long run" guideline. It keeps the workload balanced.

Variations for Interest

If you find the basic run feels repetitive, here are ways to keep it fresh while staying in Gear 2:

- **Scenery Change:** Run a different route each week: park paths, city streets, trails.

- **Companion Runs:** Invite a friend or join a group. Gear 2 pace is perfect for conversation.
- **Audio Boost:** Podcasts or audiobooks are great companions for easy runs.
- **Double-Up Days (advanced):** For higher-mileage runners, the basic run can be split into two shorter runs in one day (e.g., 30 minutes in the morning, 30 minutes in the evening).

Common Mistakes

1. **Running Too Fast:** If you can't talk comfortably, you're in Gear 3. Slow down: this is an aerobic builder, not a tempo run.
2. **Skipping Basic Runs:** Some runners think "short runs don't matter." But skipping them weakens the foundation of your training.
3. **Turning It Into Intervals:** Save your speed for designated interval days. Keep this one steady.

The Role of the Basic Run in Your Week

Think of your training week like a well-balanced meal. The long run is the main course, intervals are the spices, tempo runs are the sauce, and the basic run is the solid side dish that ties it all together. Without it, the plate feels empty.

In fact, many runners find the basic run becomes their favorite: simple, steady, no pressure — just time to move, breathe, and enjoy the rhythm of running.

◆ **Key Takeaway:** The basic run is the steady backbone of your training. It may not feel glamorous, but it quietly builds endurance, reinforces recovery, and keeps you consistent. Half the long run, all in Gear 2 — simple and powerful.

Chapter 6. The Long Interval Run (Gears 2 + 4)

If the long run builds endurance and the basic run reinforces it, the **long interval run** is where you start sharpening your fitness. By alternating between **steady Gear 2 running and harder efforts in Gear 4**, you train your body to handle sustained discomfort, recover while moving, and build speed without losing your aerobic base.

This workout is like pressing the gas pedal hard for a stretch, then easing back into cruise mode — over and over. Done right, long intervals are challenging but transformative.

Why Long Intervals Matter

1. **VO$_2$ Max Improvement:** Gear 4 efforts push your heart, lungs, and muscles close to their oxygen-using limits. Over time, this raises your "VO$_2$ max" — your maximum ability to take in and use oxygen.
2. **Lactate Tolerance:** When you run faster, your muscles produce lactate. Intervals train your body to clear lactate efficiently, so you can sustain speed longer before fatigue sets in.

3. **Speed-Endurance Bridge:** Long intervals sit between the comfort of Gear 2 and the sharpness of Gear 5. They teach you how to run faster for longer stretches — the sweet spot for 5K to half marathon racing.
4. **Mental Toughness:** Intervals teach you how to stay composed under strain, then recover and do it again. This builds confidence for race day surges, hills, or fast finishes.

Structure of a Long Interval Run

A long interval workout combines three elements:

1. **Warm-Up (10–15 minutes):** Gear 2 running, easy and relaxed. Add a few strides (10–15 seconds at faster pace) to wake up the legs.
2. **Main Set:** Alternating Gear 4 intervals with recovery, 2 minutes in Gear 1.
3. **Cool-Down (10 minutes):** Gear 2 to bring the body back to balance.

How to Run the Intervals

- **Effort Level (Gear 4):** You're working hard, breathing heavily, but still in control. Talking is possible in single words only.

- **Duration:** Each interval lasts 2–5 minutes depending on experience. 2 minutes is just fine. *Do not push past 5 minutes.*
- **Recovery:** Equal time in Gear 2. This is *active recovery* — running, not walking.

Progression Examples

Beginners

- 10 min warm-up (Gear 2)
- 3 × 1 minute in Gear 4, with 2 minutes in Gear 1 between each. Build up to 2 minutes per interval.
- 10 min cool-down (Gear 2)

Intermediate Runners

- 15 min warm-up (Gear 2)
- 4–5 × 3 minutes in Gear 4, with 2 minutes in Gear 1 between each
- 10 min cool-down (Gear 2)

More Advanced Runners

- 15 min warm-up (Gear 2)
- 5–6 × 4–5 minutes in Gear 4, with 2 minutes in Gear 1 between each.
- 10 min cool-down (Gear 2)

Tip: If you feel you could sprint at the end of each interval, you're not working hard enough. If you collapse after each one, you're going too hard. Gear 4 is tough but repeatable.

Common Mistakes

1. **Starting Too Fast:** Many runners burn out after the first interval. Start controlled, save your hardest effort for the last one.
2. **Running to fast between fast intervals**
3. **Skipping Recovery:** The Gear 2 recovery is just as important as the Gear 4 effort. It teaches your body to recover while still moving.
4. **Doing Too Many Too Soon:** Intervals are powerful but stressful. Build volume gradually.

Science in Action

Long intervals push you near your **aerobic ceiling**. Think of your lungs and heart as a pump and pipes system: the pump gets stronger, and the pipes get wider, delivering more oxygen per stride. At the same time, your muscles adapt by increasing enzymes that process oxygen, making every step more efficient.

Put simply: long intervals make your body better at turning oxygen into speed.

When to Use Long Intervals

- **Once per week** (for 4- and 5-day runners)
- **Middle of the week** works well, away from the fatigue of long runs
- **Training cycles:** Increase interval volume gradually over 6–8 weeks, then pull back during a taper before racing

---

📌 **Key Takeaway:** Long interval runs combine effort and recovery to push your aerobic engine higher. They're hard but manageable, teaching your body to run faster for longer. They are one of the most powerful tools in your training plan.

Chapter 7. The Short Interval Run (Gears 2 + 5)

If long intervals are about sustained effort, **short intervals** are about raw speed but in small, controlled doses. In the RunShift™ method, this workout blends bursts in **Gear 5** (maximum effort) with long, gentle recoveries in Neutral and Gear 1.

Short intervals may look simple on paper — a few seconds of sprinting, then lots of recovery — but don't underestimate them. These workouts teach your body to run faster, improve your stride mechanics, and boost running economy without leaving you exhausted.

Why Short Intervals Matter

1. **Neuromuscular Training:** Sprints teach your brain and muscles to communicate more efficiently, improving stride coordination and turnover.
2. **Running Economy:** By briefly hitting maximum speed, you train your body to use oxygen and energy more efficiently at *all* paces.
3. **Explosiveness:** Gear 5 recruits fast-twitch muscle fibers, which are often underused in distance running.

4. **Confidence:** Once you've sprinted all-out in training, race-day pace feels smoother and more manageable.

In short: short intervals sharpen your "engine" while keeping mileage low.

Structure of a Short Interval Run

Every short interval run follows the same flow:

1. **Warm-Up (10–15 minutes):** Gear 2 running to prepare the body. Add a few 10-second strides to wake up your legs.
2. **Main Set:** Repeated sprints (Gear 5) with 2 minutes in Gear 1 in between.
3. **Cool-Down (10 minutes):** Gear 2 running to return to balance.

The Interval Formula

Each repetition follows this structure:

- **10-20 seconds in Gear 5:** Sprint as fast as you can sustain with good form.

- **2 minutes in Gear 1 (slow jog):** Gentle reset before the next sprint. Beginners should do 1 minute in neutral followed by 1 minute in Gear 1.

That's one full cycle. Repeat the cycle several times depending on your level.

Progression Examples

Beginners

- Warm-up 10 minutes (Gear 2)
- 3 × [10s in Gear 5 + 1 min in Neutral (walk) + 1 min Gear 1]
- Cool-down 10 minutes (Gear 2)

Intermediate Runners

- Warm-up 12–15 minutes (Gear 2)
- 6 × [15s in Gear 5 + 2 min Gear 1]
- Cool-down 10 minutes (Gear 2)

More Advanced Runners

- Warm-up 15 minutes (Gear 2)
- 9 × 20s in Gear 5 + 2 min Gear 1]
- Cool-down 10 minutes (Gear 2)

Tips for Success

- **Form First:** Sprinting in poor form risks injury. Focus on tall posture, quick turnover, relaxed shoulders, and driving arms.
- **Stay Relaxed:** Don't clench fists or tense your face. Efficient sprinting comes from controlled power, not strain.
- **Leave Something in the Tank:** Sprint hard, but don't collapse at the end. The goal is repeatable efforts.
- **Shoes and Surface:** Do these on safe, flat ground with proper running shoes. Grass or track surfaces are gentler than pavement.

If you're using a heart rate monitor

If you like tracking data, your short intervals should look something like the chart below. Notice the **saw-tooth pattern**: sharp spikes upward as you sprint, followed by quick drops during recovery. This rise-and-fall cycle reflects the stress–recover rhythm that maximizes anaerobic benefit.

Aim for 3–9 of these spikes in a single session, depending on your level. Always start with a Gear 2 warm-up (take as long as you need) and finish with a Gear 2 cool-down. The warm-up prepares your muscles and heart for hard efforts, while the cool-down helps your body recover smoothly.

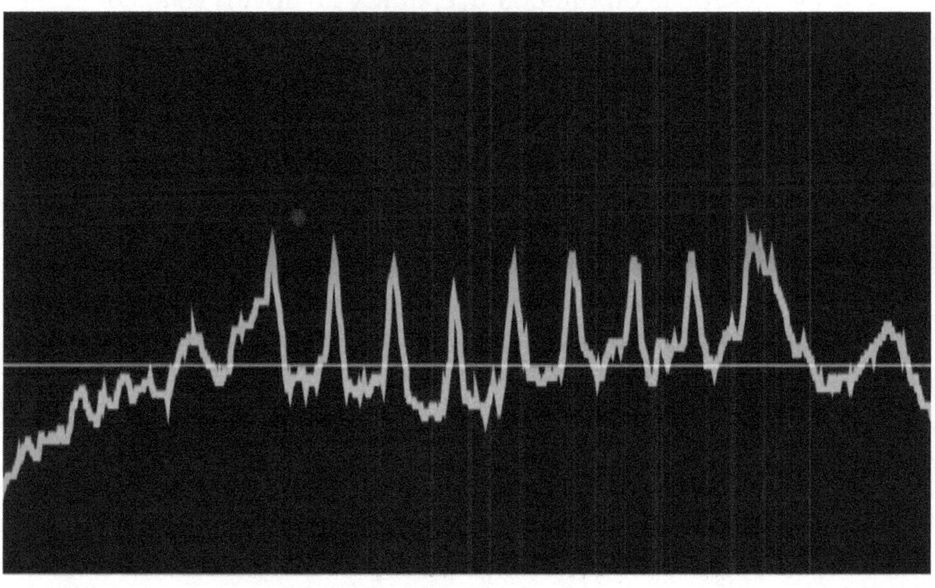

Common Mistakes

1. **Overdoing It**
   The biggest mistake is cutting recovery short. Between sprints, you should jog in **Gear 1** (very slow) for two minutes. Alternatively, you can walk

(**Neutral**) for a full minute, then jog in **Gear 1** (very slow) for one more minute. That recovery time is not wasted; it's what makes the next sprint possible. You want your heartrate to go back down as much as possible.

2. **Skipping Recovery**
   Those recoveries are essential. They allow you to hit every sprint with quality and intensity. Without them, your form breaks down, and the workout becomes less effective.

3. **Going Too Long**
   Another common slip is sprinting beyond 30 seconds. Once you pass that mark, the effort often shifts toward **Gear 4** instead of true **Gear 5.** Keep sprints short and sharp. That's the whole point.

The Science in Action

When you sprint, your body switches almost entirely to **anaerobic energy**, burning fuel without oxygen. This recruits fast-twitch muscle fibers and builds explosive strength. But the magic happens in recovery: your heartrate comes down, your breathing settles, and your aerobic system learns to reset quickly.

This "stress and recover" cycle makes you more efficient both at sprint speeds and at every pace below them. That's why even marathoners include sprints in their training.

When to Use Short Interval

- **Once per week** in a 5-day plan.
- **Every other week** in a 4-day plan (alternating with long intervals).
- **Timing:** Best done on fresh legs, not the day after a long run.

✦ **Key Takeaway:** Short intervals train raw speed, form, and efficiency. Sprint, recover generously, and repeat. Small doses of Gear 5 make every other gear feel easier.

Chapter 8. The Tempo Run (Gear 3)

If the long run is your foundation, the basic run your steady support, and intervals your sharpening tool, the **tempo run** is the bridge that ties them all together. It's the workout where you learn to run at a **"comfortably hard" pace**. This is faster than your training cruise, but not an all-out effort.

Tempo runs aren't glamorous, but they are essential. They train you to handle the kind of sustained discomfort you'll feel in the middle stages of a race, the point where the finish line still feels far away, but the pace is too fast to relax.

Why the Tempo Run Matter

1. **Raises Your Lactate Threshold:** Your muscles produce lactate at higher speeds, and if it builds up too fast, you slow down. Tempo runs train your body to clear lactate more efficiently, so you can run faster for longer.
2. **Builds Race-Day Stamina:** The tempo pace is close to your 10K or half marathon pace. Training here makes race pace feel familiar, not intimidating.
3. **Teaches Pacing Discipline:** Running "comfortably hard" without tipping into exhaustion is a skill that can make or break your race.

How a Tempo Run Feels

- **Gear:** Gear 3.
- **Talk Test:** Talking is possible only in short bursts, a few words before pausing to breathe.
- **RPE:** 6–7 out of 10.
- **Duration:** 10–40 minutes at tempo pace within the workout.

Tempo runs should feel challenging but sustainable. If you finish gasping or unable to hold the pace, you went too hard. If you could have gone on forever, you went too easy.

Structure of a Tempo Run

1. **Warm-Up (10–15 minutes):** Gear 2, easy running. Add a few strides.
2. **Main Set:** 10–20 minutes in Gear 3 for beginners, 20–30 minutes for intermediates, up to 45 minutes for more advanced runners.
3. **Cool-Down (10 minutes):** Gear 2 or Gear 1.

Example: A 5-day runner might do a 10-minute warm-up, 20 minutes in Gear 3, and a 10-minute cool-down, a solid 40-minute session.

Progression Example

- **Beginners:** 10 min warm-up → 10 min Gear 3 → 10 min cool-down in Gear 2
- **Intermediate:** 15 min warm-up → 20–25 min Gear 3 → 10 min cool-down in Gear 2
- **More Advanced:** 15 min warm-up → 35–45 min Gear 3 → 10 min cool-down in Gear 2

When to Do Tempo Run

- **4-Day Runners:** Replace your long interval run with a tempo run once per month.
- **5-Day Runners:** Include one tempo run per week.

This balance ensures you get the benefits of Gear 3 without overloading your system.

Common Mistakes

1. **Running Too Fast:** If you're gasping, you've slipped into Gear 4.
2. **Skipping Warm-Up:** Going straight into tempo pace shocks the body and raises injury risk.

3. **Doing Tempos Too Often:** They're powerful but taxing. Once per week (or less) is enough.

Key Takeaway: The tempo run is your race rehearsal: challenging but sustainable, tough but controlled. Run it in Gear 3, build pacing discipline, and learn to stay strong when running starts to feel uncomfortable.

Part II. Practical Guidance

An Important Word of Caution Before You Build and Execute Your Plan

During your runs, always listen to your body. If you experience **sharp or significant pain, dizziness, chest tightness, or unusual shortness of breath**, stop immediately and seek medical guidance. Discomfort from effort is normal; pain that feels alarming is not.

Chapter 9. Tools for Success

Running is simple at its core: shoes, open space, and your own determination. But the right tools can make your training smoother, safer, and more enjoyable. The goal is not to drown in gadgets or overcomplicate the sport; it's to use a few smart choices that support your running journey.

This chapter covers four essentials: music, watches, shoes, and hydration/fueling.

Music: Your Secret Training Partner

For many runners, music can turn a good run into a great one. The right song can lift your mood, carry you through fatigue, and help you lock into rhythm on days when the miles feel long.

My advice: create your own playlist. Make it much longer than any single run, and pack it with variety. Mix in high-energy tracks that lift you when you need a push, and calmer pieces that let you settle into rhythm. My own playlist runs over six hours, which is far more than I'll ever need, even for a marathon. And I always keep it on shuffle. That way I never know what's coming next. Sometimes a driving beat lands at the perfect moment; other times, a softer song reminds me to relax and breathe. If you want one song suggestion that captures the spirit of the RunShift™ method, try *Audience of One* by Rise Against — great beat, spot-on lyrics. But really, the key is to experiment with genres, tempos, and moods until you find the mix that makes you look forward to every run.

Of course, music isn't the only option. Some runners swear by podcasts or audiobooks. These can be great companions for easy runs, though I don't recommend highly demanding listening on interval days. Your focus and effort should be on the run itself.

📌 *Pro Tip: Building the Perfect Playlist*

- **Make it long.** Aim for a playlist much longer than any single run. That way you won't hear the same songs every session.

- **Mix it up.** Blend hard-hitting tracks that fuel intensity with calmer songs that help you find rhythm and relax.
- **Use shuffle mode.** The surprise of not knowing what comes next can give you a mental lift just when you need it.
- **Match effort to music.** Save the high-energy beats for intervals or when fatigue hits; let smoother tracks carry you through long, steady miles.
- **Test other options.** Podcasts or audiobooks can work well on easy days — but keep hard sessions music-focused so you can stay locked in.

Watches: Useful, But Don't Break the Bank

Do you need a sports watch to run well? No. Do they help? Absolutely. A sports watch can tell you your time, pace, and heartrate. These are all useful data for learning your gears.

But here's the truth: **you don't need the latest $1,000 gadget.** A simple sports watch with GPS and timing is more than enough. I've seen one-year-old models for $100–200 on resale sites, and they work perfectly for training.

Some sports watches allow you to upload custom training programs. If you have pone of those, you can upload the five training runs: basic, long, short interval, long interval and tempo, and adjust them as you improve.

RunShift™: A <u>Simple</u> 5-Gear Method for 5K, 10K, and Half Marathon Success

---

Pro Tips for Shoes

Get fitted (at least) once*: Visit a specialty running store for gait analysis. Even if you order future pairs online, that first fitting is worth it.*

Prioritize comfort*: Good shoes should disappear on your feet. Blisters, dark nails or hot spots are signs you need a different model.*

Rotate pairs*: If you run often, rotate two pairs to extend their lifespan and reduce injury risk.*

Retire on time*: Most shoes last about 500 km (300 miles). Track mileage in an app, not just appearance.*

The fancy features like wrist-based VO_2 max estimates, sleep tracking, and training load graphs are fun but not essential. Don't let tech (or marketing) convince you that you need the most expensive model to become a better runner. You don't.

Shoes: The One Item Worth Investing In

If you save money on watches, save money on music, save money on gear, that is fine by me. But **don't cut corners on shoes.**

Running shoes are the most important piece of equipment you own. The wrong shoes can lead to blisters, pain, and even injury; the right shoes feel like an extension of your body.

Ideally, visit a **specialty running store** at least once. Talk to a pro about your running style. Do you land on your heel, midfoot, or forefoot? Do you roll inward (pronate) or stay neutral? Do you need extra support (stability shoes) or a lightweight trainer?

Even if you buy future pairs online, that initial consultation is worth it. Shoes should fit not just your feet, but your gait, your mileage, and your goals.

Think of shoes as tires for a car. Good tires don't make the car faster, but they keep it safe, efficient, and enjoyable to drive.

Hydration and Fueling: Matching Effort and Climate

Water and fuel needs depend on **distance, duration, and weather.** Following current sports science, here are simple guidelines:

- **Up to 10K (under 60 minutes):** No fluids or gels needed for most people, unless it's hot and humid. In those conditions, carry water.
- **10K–20K (approx. 50–130 minutes):** Carry at least a handheld bottle of water, hydration flask, or wear a hydration backpack with a bladder. Aim to sip every 15–20 minutes. Add a gel pack every 45 minutes or so.
- **Beyond 20K (90+ minutes):** Bring water *and* energy. Take a gel or equivalent carbohydrate source about every 45 minutes. This keeps your glycogen stores topped up and prevents energy crashes.
- **Listen to your body**: Sloshing stomach or GI distress = adjust timing, type, or amount.

💡 Climate matters: In **hot, humid weather:** You'll sweat more, losing both fluids and electrolytes. In these conditions, consider electrolyte tablets or sports drinks, not just plain water. In **cool weather,** you may feel less thirsty, but don't skip fluids. Dehydration can sneak up on you even in the cold.

Practice your fueling strategy during long runs. Never wait until race day to test new gels or drinks!

Bringing It All Together

- Use **music** to make runs more enjoyable and motivating.
- Get a **watch** if you like data, but don't overspend.
- Invest in **good shoes** — they're the one essential item.
- Match **hydration and fueling** to the distance and climate.

Remember: running is about consistency, not gadgets. The right tools make it smoother, but the real progress comes from showing up, shifting through your gears, and trusting the process.

📌 **Key Takeaway:** Music keeps you inspired, a simple watch helps with pacing, shoes protect and support your body, and smart hydration fuels your runs. These are the tools that make training not just possible, but enjoyable and sustainable.

Chapter 10. Structuring Weekly Training Plans

By now, you know the gears and the workouts. But how do you put it all together into a week that makes sense? That's where structure comes in. A well-designed plan ensures you hit every system (endurance, strength, speed, and recovery) without overloading your body.

The RunShift™ method uses **4-day and 5-day weekly structures.** Both are effective. For the 5K, I also provide a **<u>3-day option</u>**. The right choice depends on your schedule, experience, and recovery needs.

In the next chapter, you'll find the 12-week training plans built using this structure. If you're eager to get started, feel free to jump straight there. In this chapter, I explain how and why the plans are structured the way they are, for readers who want to understand the reasoning behind them

Why Structure Matter

Running success comes not from one workout, but from the *balance* of workouts. Too many hard sessions and you risk burnout. Too many easy runs and you stagnate. The right structure ensures progress, consistency, and enjoyment.

Think of your training week as a balanced meal:

- The **long run** is your main dish.
- The **basic run** is your side.
- The **intervals** are your spices.
- The **tempo run** is the sauce that ties it together.

The 3/4-Day Plan

The 4-day plan is perfect for runners balancing work, family, and fitness. It includes all the essentials without overwhelming your schedule.

Weekly Flow:

- **Day 1:** Long Run (Gear 2)
- **Day 2:** Rest or active recovery
- **Day 3:** Basic Run (Gear 2, half the long run time)
- **Day 4:** Rest or cross-training
- **Day 5:** Intervals (alternate weeks: Long Intervals in Gear 4, Short Intervals in Gear 5)

- **Day 6:** Rest or walking in Neutral
- **Day 7:** Basic Run (Gear 2 steady).*

***skip for the 3-day plan.**

👉 Once per month, replace the long interval run with a **tempo run (Gear 3).**

For example, your plan could look like this:

Day	Workout	Gear Focus
Mon	Long Run	Gear 2
Tue	Rest/Recovery	
Wed	Basic Run	Gear 2
Thu	Rest/Cross	
Fri	Intervals (alternate Long/Short)	Gears 2 and 4 or 5*
Sat	Rest/Recovery	
Sun	Basic Run	Gear 2

*Once per month, replace the long interval run with a **tempo run (Gear 3).**

The 5-Day Plan

The 5-day plan includes everything in the 4-day version, plus a dedicated **tempo run** every week. This plan is ideal for runners who want more variety and are ready for an extra training load.

Weekly Flow:

- **Day 1:** Long Run (Gear 2)
- **Day 2:** Rest or active recovery
- **Day 3:** Basic Run (Gear 2, half the long run time)
- **Day 4:** Long Intervals (Gear 4)
- **Day 5:** Rest or easy recovery
- **Day 6:** Short Intervals (Gear 5)
- **Day 7:** Tempo Run (Gear 3)

For example, your plan could look like this:

Day	Workout	Gear Focus
Mon	Long Run	Gear 2
Tue	Rest/Recovery	
Wed	Basic Run	Gear 2
Thu	Long Intervals	Gears 2/4
Fri	Rest/Recovery	
Sat	Short Intervals	Gears 2/5
Sun	Tempo Run	Gears 2/3

Choosing the Right Plan

- **If you're new to structured running:** Start with the 4-day plan. It builds fitness without overwhelming your body.
- **If you're comfortable with regular training:** The 5-day plan adds intensity and variety for faster progress.
- **If life gets in the way:** Remember: missing one run is not a failure. Adjust, move forward, and stay consistent over time.

Adapting the Gears If You're Out of Shape

Before you begin, take a moment to <u>reread the note of caution</u> at the start of Chapters 1 and 9.

If you're out of shape, the RunShift Method can be adapted. Remember that it is *perfectly fine to walk in Gear 1*. If Gear 2 still doesn't feel natural, even at a very slow pace, alternate between Gears 1 and 2 during any Gear 2 interval. A simple structure works well: one minute in Gear 1 followed by one minute in Gear 2. Over time, you can increase the time spent in Gear 2 (for example, 2:1, then 3:1), but there is no need to rush.

Skip the short intervals (Gear 5) until you're comfortable with Gear 2 and replace them with a Basic Run.

The goal is to make running enjoyable and sustainable. Progress will come, and consistency matters far more than speed. You can absolutely do this.

A Word on Recovery

Rest days are not wasted days. They are when your body repairs, adapts, and grows stronger. **If you feel unusually sore, fatigued, or unmotivated, swap a workout for rest.** A consistent plan is flexible, not rigid. Avoid major cardio on those days, but consider weight training.

🔖 **Key Takeaway:** Structure keeps your training balanced. The 4-day plan builds endurance with less stress; the 5-day plan adds variety for faster progress. Choose the plan that fits your life, because the best plan is the one you can stick with.

Chapter 11. The 12-Week Training Plans

These plans are designed to take you from a solid starting point to race-ready in 12 weeks. They follow the RunShift™ principles: balance, gradual progression, and smart use of the gears.

12-Week 5K Plan (3-4 Days per Week)

Who it's for: Runners aiming to comfortably complete or improve their 5K performance.

- **Long Run:** Starts at **30 minutes** and can be extended for intermediate and advanced runners.
- **Basic Run:** Half the long run duration.
- **Intervals:** Focus on both short (Gear 5) and long (Gear 4) intervals to sharpen speed and endurance.
- **Tempo Run:** Once per month, replacing the long interval session.

A Note on Training Only Three Days per Week

If your schedule simply doesn't allow four runs per week, training three days is perfectly acceptable. You can follow the plan by skipping the second basic run and keeping the long run, one intervals session, and one basic run. Progress will still come, but it will come more slowly. With fewer runs, your body gets fewer chances to reinforce endurance and efficiency, so improvements take longer. Think of three days per week as maintenance-plus because it keeps you moving forward, just at a gentler pace. When life allows, try switching or returning to four days. It will noticeably accelerate your progress.

If the weather is warm, and especially for long runs, bring a hydration flask or water bottle.

Week	Long Run (Gear 2)	Basic Run (Gear 2)	Intervals	Basic Run #2 (Gear 2)
1	30 min	15 min	3×15s (G5)**	15 min
2	30 min	15 min	4×2 min (G4)*	15 min
3	35 min	15 min	5×15s (G5)**	20 min
4 (rec.)	25 min	15 min	3×15s (G5)**	15 min
5	35 min	20 min	5×2 min (G4)*	20 min
6	40 min	20 min	6×15s (G5)**	20 min
7	40 min	20 min	Tempo Run 15m	20 min

RunShift™: A <u>Simple</u> 5-Gear Method for 5K, 10K, and Half Marathon Success

Week	Long Run (Gear 2)	Basic Run (Gear 2)	Intervals	Basic Run #2 (Gear 2)
8 (rec.)	30 min	15 min	4×15s (G5)**	15 min
9	40 min	20 min	6×2 min (G4)*	20 min
10	45 min	20 min	7×15s (G5)**	25 min
11	45 min	25 min	Tempo Run 20m	25 min
12 (taper)	30 min	15 min	3×15s (G5)**	15 min

* For long intervals, 2 minutes in Gear 1 between each

** For short intervals, 2 minutes in Gear 1 between each. Beginners should walk (neutral) for one minute and then do one minute in Gear 1 between each.

Key Takeaway for 5K Runners:

- Beginners: stick to the minimums listed.
- Intermediate: extend the long run to 40–50 minutes.
- More advanced runners can extend the long run up to 60 minutes if preparing for a faster 5K.

12-Week 10K Plan (4-5 Days per Week)

Who it's for: Runners aiming to comfortably complete or improve at the 10K distance.

- **Long Run:** Starts at **55 minutes** and can be extended for more experienced runners.
- **Basic Run:** About half the long run duration.
- **Long Intervals:** Gear 4 efforts to build speed endurance.
- **Short Intervals:** Gear 5 sprints for sharpness.
- **Tempo Runs:** Weekly, 15–30 minutes in Gear 3.

Week	Long Run[a] (Gear 2)	Basic Run (Gear 2)	Long Intervals* (Gear 4)	Short Intervals** (Gear 5)	Tempo Run (Gear 3)
1	55 min	25 min	3×2 min	3×15s	15 min
2	60 min	30 min	4×3 min	4×15s	20 min
3	70 min	35 min	5×3 min	5×15s	20 min
4 (rec.)	50 min	25 min	3×2 min	3×15s	15 min
5	75 min	35 min	4×4 min	5×15s	25 min

RunShift™: A <u>Simple</u> 5-Gear Method for 5K, 10K, and Half Marathon Success

Week	Long Run[a] (Gear 2)	Basic Run (Gear 2)	Long Intervals* (Gear 4)	Short Intervals** (Gear 5)	Tempo Run (Gear 3)
6	80 min	40 min	5×4 min	6×15s	25 min
7	85 min	40 min	6×4 min	7×15s	30 min
8 (rec.)	60 min	30 min	3×3 min	4×15s	20 min
9	85 min	40 min	6×5 min	7×15s	30 min
10	90 min	45 min	5×5 min	8×15s	30 min
11	90 min	45 min	6×5 min	9×15s	30 min
12 (taper***)	60 min	30 min	3×3 min	3×15s	20 min

* *a*: For long runs, bringing hydration (water with or without electrolytes) and a gel pack is advisable, two if you plan to run more than 90 minutes.

* For long intervals, 2 minutes in Gear 1 between each

** For short intervals, 2 minutes in Gear 1 between each. Beginners should walk (neutral) for one minute and then do one minute in Gear 1 between each.

***In taper week (before a race), I recommend taking two or three days before race day *off*; if you do choose to run, keep it short and easy.

👉 **Note:** Long run times below are **minimum recommendations.** If you're intermediate, extend your long run by 5–10 minutes. Advanced runners can extend up to 100 minutes as long as the pace stays in **Gear 2.**

12-Week Half Marathon Plan (5 Days per Week)

Who it's for: Runners aiming to complete or improve at the half marathon distance.

- **Long Run:** Starts at **60 minutes** and builds toward 120 minutes.
- **Basic Run:** About half the long run.
- **Intervals:** Weekly sessions in Gears 4 and 5.
- **Tempo Runs:** Weekly, 20–40 minutes in Gear 3.

👉 **Note:** These long run times are **minimums**.

- **Intermediate runners** can extend by 15 minutes.

- **More advanced runners** may build beyond 2 hours, but should do so very gradually, with plenty of recovery, and always in **Gear 2.**

Week	Long Run[a] (Gear 2)	Basic Run (Gear 2)	Long Intervals* (Gear 4)	Short Intervals** (Gear 5)	Tempo Run (Gear 3)
1	60 min	30 min	3×3 min	3×15s	20 min
2	70 min	35 min	4×3 min	4×15s	25 min
3	80 min	40 min	5×3 min	5×15s	25 min
4 (rec.)	60 min	30 min	3×2 min	3×15s	20 min
5	90 min	45 min	4×4 min	5×15s	30 min
6	100 min	50 min	5×4 min	6×15s	30 min
7	110 min	55 min	6×4 min	7×15s	35 min
8 (rec.)	75 min	40 min	3×3 min	4×15s	25 min
9	100 min	50 min	5×5 min	6×15s	35 min
10	110 min	55 min	6×5 min	7×15s	35 min

Week	Long Run[a] (Gear 2)	Basic Run (Gear 2)	Long Intervals* (Gear 4)	Short Intervals** (Gear 5)	Tempo Run (Gear 3)
11	120 min	60 min	6×5 min	9×15s	40 min
12 (taper***)	60 min	30 min	3×3 min	3×15s	---------

a: For long runs, bringing hydration (water with or without electrolytes) and a gel pack (after 45 minutes) is advisable; two if running more than 90 minutes.

* For long intervals, 2 minutes in Gear 1 between each

** For short intervals, 2 minutes in Gear 1 between each.

***In taper week (before a race), I recommend taking two or three days before race day *off*; if you do choose to run, keep it short and easy.

How to Use These Plans

- **Consistency beats perfection.** Missing a session here and there is normal. Just move forward.
- **Respect recovery weeks.** Every fourth week, runs are shorter. That's when your body absorbs training.

- **Adapt as needed.** If you feel too fatigued, reduce interval volume or pace. The gears are flexible tools, not rigid demands.

- 📌 **Key Takeaways:** These 12-week plans give you a clear roadmap. Whether you're training for a 5K, 10K, or half marathon, the RunShift™ method balances gears, builds endurance, and prepares you for race day. The long runs listed are **starting points**. Beginners should stick to the minimums.
- Intermediate runners should extend moderately.
- Advanced runners can add time to build extra endurance, but only if they stay in **Gear 2** and allow proper recovery.

Chapter 12. The Mental Side of RunShift™

Running is not just a physical act. It's mental. Ask ultramarathoners and they will tell you that success is 90% in the mind. The long run tests your patience, the tempo run tests your discipline, and intervals test your willingness to push into discomfort. To thrive as a runner, you need to train not only your legs and lungs, but also your mindset. Running is not only physical; it resonates with something deep in our evolutionary wiring. Perhaps that's why many runners describe long runs as meditative: we're doing what humans have done for thousands of years.

Consistency Over Motivation

Many runners wait for motivation to strike before lacing up. The truth is, motivation is fleeting. Discipline is what gets you out the door on cold mornings or busy evenings.

Think of your runs as **appointments with yourself.** You wouldn't cancel a meeting with your boss or your doctor. Treat your runs with the same respect. Motivation will come and go, but consistency builds habits, and habits build results.

Breaking the Run into Chunks

One of the best mental tricks is to divide a run into smaller parts:

- **For long runs:** Think of them as "three 20-minute runs" rather than one 60-minute grind.
- **For tempo runs:** Focus on getting through the first 5 minutes, then reset your mind.
- **For intervals:** Concentrate only on the next rep, never the whole workout at once.

By shrinking the challenge, you reduce mental fatigue and stay present.

Mind Spotlight: Running as Moving Meditation

Modern science suggests that running doesn't just train your body; it taps into ancient mental pathways. For early humans, endurance running wasn't optional. Covering long distances together required focus, rhythm, and calm persistence. Those who could stay steady under discomfort — physically and mentally — were the ones who endured.

Today, many runners describe long runs as meditative. That isn't an accident:

Rhythm and breath calm the nervous system, much like controlled breathing in meditation.

Repetition lets the mind settle, making space for reflection and problem-solving.

Connection to nature echoes the landscapes our ancestors once crossed.

Flow state: Neuroscience shows that repetitive endurance exercise can trigger flow, a state of focused ease that feels deeply restorative.

When you settle into Gear 2, you're not just training your body's endurance engine. You're practicing the same mental resilience and rhythm that helped our species survive. Running becomes more than exercise. It becomes a way of returning to something

Learning to Be Comfortable with Discomfort

Running is supposed to feel challenging sometimes. The key is knowing the difference between *good discomfort* (lungs burning, legs heavy, but body under control) and *bad pain* (sharp, stabbing, or worsening).

- **Good discomfort:** Builds resilience. Stay with it.
- **Bad pain:** A warning sign. Stop immediately.

Trust yourself to know the difference. Training teaches not only endurance but also awareness of your own body.

Visualization and Positive Self-Talk

Elite runners often visualize their races in advance, picturing the course, the effort, even the finish line. You can use the same tool in training: imagine yourself running strong, relaxed, and confident.

Equally powerful is **self-talk.** Replace thoughts like *"I can't hold this"* with *"One more minute, then I decide."* Or *"I'm strong, I've done this before, I can do it again."* Your inner voice should become your most loyal training partner... nor your harshest critic. Choose wisely.

The Role of Rest and Recovery

A strong mindset isn't about pushing endlessly. It's about knowing when to pull back. Listening to your body, taking a rest day when needed, or swapping a hard session for an easy one is not weakness. It's wisdom.

Think of it this way: your body gets stronger during recovery, not during the run itself. Training breaks you down. Recovery builds you up. A disciplined runner respects both sides of the process.

Race-Day Nerves and Focus

Even experienced runners feel nervous before races. That's normal: it means you care. Use nerves to your advantage by channeling them into focus.

- Stick to your gears. Don't start too fast.
- Use the **talk test** or RPE to stay in the right effort.
- Remind yourself: *I've trained for this. I know my gears. I belong here.*

Running as Community

Running can be an amazing solitary meditation when it's just you and the road, but it can also be a deeply social act. Our ancestors ran together for survival, for food, for migration. Today, we can still form bonds through the miles we share. Modern running clubs, group long runs, and even the unspoken nod between strangers on a trail all remind us that running connects us. The rhythm of footsteps side by side builds trust and companionship in a way few other activities can. Whether you train with a partner, join a weekend group, or line up at a race surrounded by thousands, running reminds you that progress isn't only individual; it's something you can share.

Running Together

Running may feel like a solo sport, and it can be, but it can also be social.

- ***Shared rhythm:*** *Running side by side builds trust and companionship.*
- ***Modern tribes:*** *Clubs, park runs, and race-day crowds recreate the communal energy of our ancestors running together.*
- ***Motivation boost:*** *Training partners keep you accountable, and even a silent nod to a fellow runner can lift your spirits.*

The mental benefits of running multiply when we share the miles. Every stride reminds us that progress is not just individual; it's something we can create together.

Key Takeaway: The mental side of running is about discipline, patience, and perspective. Break challenges into smaller pieces, embrace good discomfort, use positive self-talk, and respect recovery. Training your mind is training your body — they grow stronger together.

Chapter 13. Racing with Gears

Training teaches you how to shift gears. Racing is where you put that skill into practice. A good race isn't about going all-out from the start; it's about knowing when to stay steady, when to push, and when to unleash what you've trained for.

The RunShift™ method gives you a simple framework: treat your race like driving a car with a manual transmission. Start smooth, shift up gradually, and finish strong.

General Principles for Any Race

1. **Don't Burn Out Early:** Many runners sprint off the start line, only to fade badly later. Hold back. Start in control.
2. **Run Your Own Race:** Stick to your gears, not the pace of others. Let them go if they're too fast. You'll catch them later.
3. **Trust Your Training:** You've practiced your gears for weeks. Race day is about executing what you already know.
4. **Use Mental Landmarks:** Break the race into sections. Don't think "I have 10K left"; think "just hold Gear 2 for the next 10 minutes."

The 5K: Fast and Focused

The 5K is short, but it's still a race that rewards smart pacing. For your first 5K, you are just establishing a baseline. To do this:

- **Start (0–1 km / 0–0.5 mi):** Begin in **Gear 2.** Adrenaline is high. Don't waste it by sprinting.
- **Middle (1–4 km / 0.5–2.5 mi):** Shift into **Gear 3.** This is your tempo effort: tough but controlled.
- **Final Push (last km / last 0.5 mi):** Shift into **Gear 4.** If you have something left in the tank, unleash a brief **Gear 5 sprint** to the finish.

Mental Tip: Remind yourself the discomfort is short-lived. A 5K is over quickly so stay brave in Gear 3.

The 10K: A Test of Patience

The 10K doubles the distance of the 5K but more than doubles the mental challenge. Go out too fast and the second half becomes a struggle. For your first 10K, you are just establishing a baseline. To do this:

- **Start (0–2 km / 0–1.5 mi):** Begin in **Gear 2.** It will feel too easy, that's good.

- **Middle (2–7 km / 1.5–4.5 mi):** Hold steady in **Gear 3.** This is your main racing gear.
- **Final Push (last 3 km / 1.5–2 mi):** Shift to **Gear 4.** If you have reserves, finish the final stretch with a surge into **Gear 5.**

Mental Tip: Think of the race in *two halves*. The first half is control; the second half is courage.

The Half Marathon: Endurance and Resilience

The half marathon is long enough to demand patience, but short enough that pacing mistakes still hurt. This is where gears really shine.

For your first half-marathon, stick to Gear 2. The idea is to finish and establish a baseline. If this is your first, by definition you will have a new "PR!" The structure I recommend once you're level allows is to aim for something like this:

- **Start (0–5 km / 0–3 mi):** Run in **Gear 2.** This should feel steady and almost "too easy." Save your energy.
- **Middle (5–15 km / 3–9 mi):** Shift into **Gear 3.** This is your sustainable race gear. Talking in short bursts only.

- **Late Race (15–19 km / 9–12 mi):** Stay in **Gear 3,** but mentally prepare to push harder.
- **Final Push (last 2 km / 1 mi):** If you have anything left, shift into **Gear 4.**

Pro Tip: Mentally divide the half marathon into thirds (approximately 4.3 mi / 7km miles each):

- First third: *Patience.*
- Second third: *Control.*
- Final third: *Determination.*

Fueling and Gear Management on Race Day

- **5K/10K:** Usually no fueling needed unless conditions are hot. Just hydrate well beforehand and immediately after.
- **Half Marathon:** Start well hydrated, sip water at aid stations, and take a gel every 45 minutes if you've practiced this in training. I find it helpful to take a gel just before the race.

Always race in the **shoes and gear you've trained with.** Never try something new on race day.

Using Music for Racing

If you train with music, consider using it on race day, especially if you're running alone. Build a playlist that mirrors your race strategy:

- Easy, steady songs for the start.
- Energizing beats for the middle.
- Hard-hitting tracks for the final push.

Or shuffle it, like I do, for surprise boosts along the way.

The Community of Racing

On race day, the miles are yours to run, but you're never running alone. From the nervous chatter at the start line to the cheers along the course and the final push toward the finish, racing turns an individual effort into a collective experience. The shared energy of thousands of footsteps can carry you further than you thought possible. Every race is proof that running is more than a sport; it's a community moving forward together.

Common Race-Day Mistakes

1. **Starting Too Fast:** The most common error at every distance. Stick to Gear 2 early.

2. **Ignoring Gears:** Don't let nerves push you off-plan. Trust your system.
3. **Skipping Fuel/Hydration:** Especially critical in the half marathon.
4. **New Gear on Race Day:** No new shoes, watches, or supplements. Stick to what you know.

◆ **Key Takeaway:** Racing with gears gives you control. Start steady, shift up gradually, and finish strong. Whether it's a 5K, 10K, or half marathon, the RunShift™ method helps you run smarter — and enjoy the race more.

Chapter 14. Testimonials

The RunShift™ method isn't just theory; it's been tested in real lives, by real runners. Here are condensed stories from people I met over the years who used the gears to change the way they train, race, and even think about running.

Daphne: From Beginner to 10K Finisher

Daphne, 32, had never thought of herself as a "runner." She started by mixing walking with Gear 1 jogging, always reminding herself that Neutral and Gear 1 had value. Within a few weeks, she was running 20 minutes without stopping. She's the friend mentioned in the preface who said that RunShift™ was "simple enough to follow and powerful enough to work." I could not have said it better myself.

The breakthrough came when she understood **Gear 2**: steady, comfortable, not too fast. That became her training sweet spot. Bit by bit, her long runs grew from 20 minutes to 60.

Three months later, Daphne crossed the finish line of her first 10K — strong, smiling, and proud. "Before, I thought running was about going as hard as you can. Now I know it's about finding the right gear and staying patient," she said.

Maya: From the Gym to Half Marathoner

I will let Maya tell you her story: "I always thought I was fit. I lift weights five days a week and did cardio at the gym. But whenever I tried to run, I'd burn out before finishing a 5K. It was frustrating because I felt strong, but running never clicked. Then I found JJ and his RunShift Method™. Learning to train in gears completely changed everything. Starting in Gear 2 made running feel manageable, and gradually shifting up built my endurance without leaving me wrecked. Now, at 23, I've finished three half marathons, something I never imagined possible. Running has gone from being my weakness to one of the things I'm most proud of."

Pierre: Cutting 14 Minutes Off a Half Marathon PR

Pierre, 41, was an experienced runner stuck at a plateau. No matter how hard he trained, he couldn't beat his half marathon personal record. His problem? Too much time in high gears.

With RunShift™, Pierre learned to spend most of his training in **Gear 2** instead of pushing every run. He used **tempo runs in Gear 3** wisely to build stamina and **intervals in Gear 4** to sharpen his speed.

In 12 weeks, Pierre not only felt stronger in training; he ran a new half marathon PR, finishing 13 minutes and 55 seconds faster. "I used to think running faster meant running hard all the time. Now I see that recovery in the lower gears makes the higher gears possible," he told me. I was just as proud as he was.

Sophie: Building Endurance Without Injury

At 62, Sophie wanted to enjoy running but feared getting injured. She had seen friends sidelined by shin splints, knees, or hips. The gears gave her a framework to train safely.

She spent most of her time in **Gear 1 and Gear 2**, learning to enjoy easy running and long walks. Every week she added just a few minutes to her long run. The result? Endurance without strain.

Six months later, Sophie was running comfortably for over an hour, something she never thought possible. And most importantly, she did it **injury-free.** "The gears gave me permission to go slow. That made running joyful, not painful," she said.

Eleanor: From 1 minute to 5K Finisher

At 38, Eleanor described herself as "unable to run even a minute." Carrying extra weight, she felt self-conscious and discouraged. The RunShift Method™ changed that by breaking progress into small, manageable steps. She began in Gear 1, walking short intervals, and moved through the gears *at her own pace.* Because RunShift is not about specific paces, she learned that even walking counted as real training.

Week by week, her endurance grew. Twelve weeks later, Eleanor completed her first 5K in just over 40 minutes. For her, the victory wasn't the time; it was running every step. "The gears made it feel possible. Every week I just shifted up a little more. Now I feel like a runner," she said.

The Power of the Gears

Each of these runners had different goals and challenges. But the gears gave them a shared language and a roadmap: start easy, build steadily, and shift with purpose. Whether you're chasing a personal best, avoiding injury, or just starting out, the gears meet you where you are… and take you where you want to go.

🔖 **Key Takeaway:** Real runners — beginner, intermediate, older, and starting from scratch — all succeeded by trusting the gears. Whatever your background, the RunShift™ method adapts to you.

Chapter 15. The Future of Your Running

By now, you've learned the gears, practiced the workouts, and seen how a structured plan can transform your running. But finishing a race or completing a training cycle is not the end; it's just the beginning. The real reward of RunShift™ is discovering a way to run that you can sustain for life.

Beyond the First Goal

Maybe your first goal was to complete a 5K, a 10K, or even a half marathon. Once you achieve it, you'll naturally ask: *What's next?*

- Some runners decide to improve their times.
- Others extend their distance.
- Many simply enjoy staying active, healthy, and consistent.

Whatever you choose, the gears give you a framework that adapts to your ambitions. They are as useful for maintaining health in your sixties as they are for chasing a new personal best in your thirties.

Building on Your Base

The aerobic foundation you've built in **Gear 2** doesn't vanish when your training cycle ends. In fact, it gets stronger with time and consistency.

Keep running 3–4 days per week in Gear 2, sprinkle in intervals or tempos when you want a challenge, and continue the long run once a week. This balance maintains your fitness and leaves you ready for any new challenge.

Cross-Training for Balance

Running is powerful, but it isn't everything. Adding other activities can make you stronger and more resilient:

- **Cycling or Swimming:** Boost cardiovascular fitness without pounding the joints.
- **Strength Training:** Builds muscle to support knees, hips, and core stability.
- **Yoga or Mobility Work:** Enhances flexibility, posture, and recovery.

Cross-training keeps your body balanced and lowers injury risk. Think of it as shifting into another kind of gear that supports your running by working different systems. I do strength training on recovery days.

Staying Motivated Long-Term

Motivation will ebb and flow. Here are a few ways to keep running fresh:

- **Set New Challenges:** Try a trail race, a new distance, or a fun run in another city, or sign up for big race a few months away.
- **Run with Others:** Join a club, find a running buddy, or enter charity races.
- **Celebrate Small Wins:** A new weekly mileage record, an interval workout finished strong, or even just consistency over a busy month.

RunShift™ works because it's flexible. Some weeks you'll do all your runs. Other weeks, life will get in the way. That's normal. What matters is getting back into your gears, again and again.

Running for Life

Running is more than training plans and races. It's fresh air in your lungs, rhythm in your stride, and clarity in your mind. It's health, confidence, and the simple joy of movement.

The gears give you structure, but they also give you freedom: freedom to run easy when you want to recover, to push when you feel strong, and to progress at your own pace.

Key Takeaway: RunShift™ isn't just about finishing a program. It's about building a sustainable, lifelong relationship with running. With gears as your guide, you can run smarter, safer, and more joyfully — for as long as you want.

Epilogue: Shifting Forward

Running is never just about miles or minutes. It's about rhythm, patience, resilience, and the quiet victories that build over time. The RunShift™ method gives you more than a training plan; **it gives you a clear language for your inner conversation as you run**, a way to understand effort, to listen to your body, and to know when to hold back and when to push.

The gears are simple, but their impact is powerful. Neutral reminds you that rest is part of progress. Gears 1 and 2 build your foundation. Gear 3 teaches resilience, Gear 4 adds strength, and Gear 5 brings sharpness. Together, they form a method you can carry into every run, every race, every season of your running life.

Whatever your goal (finishing your first 5K, chasing a personal best, or simply running for the joy of it), the gears are yours to use, adapt, and master.

So lace up. Find your rhythm. Shift when you need to. And remember: Running doesn't end with a finish line; it shifts with you through life.

- In one season, you may push new distances.
- In another, you may focus on staying consistent.
- Sometimes, the win is simply putting on your shoes.

The RunShift Method™ adapts at every stage. Every run is a chance to shift forward — toward strength, freedom, and the runner you were meant to be.

A Note from the Author

Thank you for reading *RunShift™*. I hope this guide has given you a clear, simple way to enjoy running more and to train with confidence.

If you found this book helpful, I would be truly grateful if you could take a minute to leave a review on Amazon. Reviews make a huge difference: they help other runners discover the book and decide if it's right for them.

Your feedback also helps me keep improving. Whether it's one sentence or a full reflection, every review matters.

👉 On Kindle, you'll see a prompt at the end of the book. Just click and share your thoughts.

Thank you for being part of the running community and for supporting this project. Wishing you many strong, joyful miles ahead.

— JJ Archer

Appendices

Appendix A: Training Plan Charts at a Glance

3/4-Day Weekly Structure

- **Day 1:** Long Run (Gear 2)
- **Day 2:** Rest or Active Recovery
- **Day 3:** Basic Run (Gear 2, half the long run)
- **Day 4:** Rest or Cross-Training
- **Day 5:** Intervals (alternate Long/Short)
- **Day 6:** Rest or Neutral (walking/light jog)
- **Day 7:** Basic Run (Gear 2 steady) (skip for 3 day)

👉 Once per month, replace Long Intervals with a Tempo Run.

5-Day Weekly Structure

- **Day 1:** Long Run (Gear 2)
- **Day 2:** Rest or Active Recovery
- **Day 3:** Basic Run (Gear 2, half the long run)
- **Day 4:** Long Intervals (Gear 4)
- **Day 5:** Rest or Recovery
- **Day 6:** Short Intervals (Gear 5)
- **Day 7:** Tempo Run (Gear 3)

12-Week Plans Overview

- **5K Plan:** Long runs 30–45 min (extend up to 60 min for advanced).
- **10K Plan:** Long runs 55–90 min (extend up to 100 min for advanced).
- **Half Marathon Plan:** Long runs 60–120 min (extend beyond 2 hours cautiously if advanced).

Appendix B: Fueling and Hydration Quick Guide

- **Up to 10K (under 60 min):** Sip water if hot/humid.
- **10K–20K (60–120 min):** Carry a handheld bottle or hydration pack. Sip every 15–20 minutes.
- **Beyond 20K (90+ min):** Add fuel. Take a gel or 30–60g carbs/hour every 45 minutes.
- **Hot/Humid Weather:** Prioritize electrolytes (sports drink or tablets).
- **Cool Weather:** Thirst signals may be weaker so drink proactively but avoid overhydration.

Appendix C: Glossary of Key Terms

- **Gear:** A running effort zone based on comfort, breathing, and sustainability.
- **Long Run:** The longest run of the week, always in Gear 2.
- **Basic Run:** Half the long run, steady in Gear 2.
- **Interval Run:** Alternating hard effort (Gear 4 or 5) with recovery.
- **Tempo Run:** A sustained effort in Gear 3, "comfortably hard."
- **Neutral:** Walking or very light movement for recovery.
- **RPE:** Rate of Perceived Exertion, a 1–10 scale of effort.
- **Talk Test:** Simple method to judge running effort by conversation ability.
- **VO$_2$ Max:** Maximum oxygen your body can use during intense exercise.
- **Lactate Threshold:** The effort level where fatigue chemicals build up faster than your body can clear them.

Appendix D: Resources and Recommended Reading

- Books & Articles
  - Jack Daniels, *Daniels' Running Formula* — science of training zones.
  - Matt Fitzgerald, *80/20 Running* — importance of easy running.
  - Deena Kastor, *Let Your Mind Run* — mental strategies from an Olympian.
  - Dennis M. Bramble & Daniel E. Lieberman, <u>Endurance running and the evolution of Homo</u> (2004) Nature 432: 345–352.
- Apps & Tools
  - Strava (tracking & community)
  - Garmin Connect (GPS data, free training plans); Polar; Apple
  - Nike Run Club (beginner-friendly guidance)